THRIVE WITH LGL-LEUKEMIA
AND AUTOIMMUNE,
NOT JUST SURVIVE

by

Dr. Sage Campione, DC

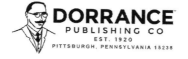

DORRANCE
PUBLISHING CO
EST. 1920
PITTSBURGH, PENNSYLVANIA 15238

The contents of this work, including, but not limited to, the accuracy of events, people, and places depicted; opinions expressed; permission to use previously published materials included; and any advice given or actions advocated are solely the responsibility of the author, who assumes all liability for said work and indemnifies the publisher against any claims stemming from publication of the work.

Disclaimer

This book contains advice and information relating to health and is not meant to diagnose, treat, or prescribe. It should be used to supplement rather than replace the advice of your physician or other trained health-care practitioner. If you know or suspect you have a medical condition, have physical symptoms, or feel unwell, seek your physician's advice before embarking on any medical program or treatment. All efforts have been made to assure the accuracy of the information contained in this book as of the date of its publication. The author does not accept any responsibility for your health, how you choose to use the information contained in this book, or your medical outcomes resulting from applying the methods suggested in this book. This is strictly the author's story and the methods she implemented to achieve better health due to her circumstances.

Dorrance Publishing Co
585 Alpha Drive
Pittsburgh, PA 15238
Visit our website at www.dorrancebookstore.com

ISBN: 978-1-6853-7341-2
eISBN: 978-1-6853-7657-4

To my mother,
she was my best cheerleader.

And to my husband,
who loved me through this all.

Very practical information with useful tips on living healthy, to thrive with this disease.

– Dr. Antonio Moran, Jr. MD, FACP

I really appreciate Dr. Sage Campione's message 'optimize your health and take care of yourself'.

– Dr. Thomas P. Loughran Jr., MD
University of Virginia

FORWARD

This book is not by a casual observer of dis-ease, autoimmune, or leukemia, but by an actual practitioner who has personally walked her path to health and advised thousands of patients to find their path too. For that reason, it is personal, practical, and easily understood. In my opinion, it is the best existing personal walk on the subject.

I first met Dr. Sage Campione in 2013 as a patient. She helped me to navigate peri-menopause. At that time, she was speaking a language that very few understood. After listening and digging deep, we discovered that I had Hashimoto Thyroiditis, but I was not experiencing symptoms at that time. Hashimoto's Thyroiditis, Rheumatoid Arthritis, and Lupus are all Auto-Immune Diseases. They attack certain organs or multiple organs but each is a disorder of the immune system. When an autoimmune disease occurs in women, during life changes it is misdiagnosed as a hormonal problem. Through that discovery, she was able to give me the tools to manage my disease so that it would not hijack my life. It was the most productive time that I had ever spent with a practitioner with the most desired results. She engaged me in being proactive and working with her on "My Team" to put the pieces together in helping me to be strong and vital, as possible. I was changing careers and just finished courses in nutritional counseling. She was authentically delighted that I was entering the field of nutrition and supportive of my goals. When we finished our work together as a doctor/patient relationship, Dr. Sage invited me to be a part of her work team. In the years since I have seen Dr. Sage's passion for what she does and her thirst for knowledge in this ever-changing field. Her commitment to her craft is evident, she is always engaging in education, webinars, conferences, and research keeping current on new and cutting-edge trends. She has been a wonderful mentor and I am always amazed and inspired by her dedication to supporting me and our patients. Through the years, Dr. Sage has had her own health challenges, including a very serious episode last year with covid. I witnessed her utilizing all of her knowledge and her faith to cure her post covid issues. I believe that she recovered her total health, which now enables her to live a more vital life.

For those of you that do not know, Dr. Sage is progressive and aggressive with her health. She is challenged by her health condition yet her nickname is 'detective' because she will grit into the issue and she is determined to find a solution. That tenacity is also how she cares for her patients.

I am so proud to call her my friend & colleague and I am grateful to have been a witness to her journey because it only confirms that she is on the right path, and a champion to have in your corner.

With Love,
Jill Shanahan, Lifestyle Specialist

A Functional Nutritionist and Mind/Body Coach, Jill has been working alongside Dr. Sage Campione in her practice; Concierge Wellness Care for 9 years. Jill writes blogs, and newsletters and consults remotely with Telehealth for the practice. She and her husband reside in Florida. She is passionate about fitness, family, and music

CONTENTS

PROLOGUE

This book was written to give you hope, to let you know there are choices, and to give you a better understanding of your health crisis. I have been living with LGLL since 2011. In the last four years, I have acquired Hemolytic Anemia. I need blood transfusions every 7 weeks. I do not take any medication. Yet, I need desforal in an IV 2x a week to keep my Ferritin levels manageable. Sometimes LGL is quiet in my life, and then there are times, it is all I think about in and out of the doctor's office. I believe it wax and wanes, like life. If I am in crisis, stressed, or something terrible is happening unexpected, then my LGL becomes a problem I need to focus on. I strongly recommend finding one or two health advocates that hear you, listen, encourage, and support you. The rest of the world is too busy; too caught up in quick fixes; too superficial. Whether you are a reflective person or an expressive person, find your healthy outlets, take notes, slow down, and breathe.

I will give you steps to take to thrive in your health. Begin now by searching for the best Integrative Practitioner to add to your health team to advise and support you in your walk. A great resource is the

University of Arizona College of Integrative Medicine. I will offer suggestions and share what I personally did to help my health. You choose with your Practitioner what will work for you. Choose wisely. Yet, please do something to help yourself.

Although we are all different, we are part of this 2 percent family of LGLL. We share this disorder, and so, we are connected.

1

DIAGNOSIS: LGL LEUKEMIA (BIG DEAL)

Oh, do not get me wrong—the first news of this diagnosis is riveting through the body. Shock, denial, a thunder and lightning of fear, and a flash of everything going on in your life, all happens in what feels like hours, yet it was only a minute. It is a horrible diagnosis for anyone to hear. Let's just focus on it. They refer you to a hematologist, who studies blood disorders, which happens to be an oncologist (CANCER) doctor's office. That alone is unnerving. Questions in your mind, like, *This cannot be for me—this must be for another family member, I am too young, I have things I want to still do in life...* All these thoughts just race through your mind, denial at its best. It is completely normal. First of all, only in Unites States do they lop these two professions in one office. In Europe, for example, hematologists have their own practice. You have a blood condition. Hear this and know this.

Although you will die with LGL Leukemia, you will not die from it. This is not a death sentence. It will be a journey of you getting to know your body and your limitations. It is an unfortunate condition because it compromises your life and oftentimes can reroute your plans. This book is to inform and encourage you that it is okay; you will manage and manage greatly by following a personal supportive health protocol.

Going forward, do not be intimated by doctors. The information they have is all they have to give. It is up to you to truly listen and hear your own body. I am often told by Dr. Antonio Moran, my local Hematologist, "You are just kicking the can, waiting for science to catch up to you to find a cure". From now on, wherever you are on this journey, keep records and copies of your blood labs, exams, and diagnostics. Keep a log of medications and how they affected you and how your body responded. Be proactive. You will find ultimately you need to care because no one will care to the depths of your concern. I care; I am in it along with you. We are only a few in this world, but we share this condition, and no one seems to explain to us why we have this condition.

2
LAB WORK

It is very important to have a detailed lab work of your WBCs. Try to maintain all copies of your labs and keep a hard copy at your home in a file marked medical; date the file by year. It is important to see if your levels are getting worse or better. It is also very important to have more detailed labs ordered. LGL directly affects our neutrophils, which are a component of the WBCs. Yet reviewing your WBC differential will help you stay aware of your LGL. I also recommend lymphocytes by Cyrex labs. Once you have these results, you will have a better idea of your overall immune system. This test is the most comprehensive look at what cells are being affected, and this will also confirm the nature of your autoimmune. The lab test will give you a deeper look into T-cells, B cells, and natural killer cells (or NK). These cells are critical to have plenty. They are your natural killer cells, and keep viral infections in check. They are the initial defense against pathogens, and they are part of our innate immune system. I have had a similar test taken at Mayo, but it was 200 percent more costly, and I found Cyrex lab test to be more helpful for me.

These are not the only labs available to us. I chose to understand 'why'. I wanted to know why I have this disease, leukemia. I started researching labs. Since, these tests are not covered by insurance I wanted to choose wisely. I first tested my nutrition levels. I discovered that my B-vitamins and my antioxidants were very low. Actually, they were too low. My glutathione level was almost insignificant. Glutathione is a major antioxidant. A huge protector against cancer and fights free radicals that cause damage to our cells. It also can repair DNA and regulate our immune system. My next step was to find out why would my glutathione be so low, how long has it been low, and how do I increase my glutathione. I decided to test my Oxidative Stress Markers. This lab by Genova Diagnostics measures; Glutathione, Lipid Peroxides, 8-OHdG, and Coenzyme Q10, ubiquinone. I discovered the two toxins; Lipid Peroxidase and 8-OHdG were very elevated. I was not breaking down my toxins like a normal person. My body was actually storing toxins and they were causing severe damage to my cells. So, I tested for toxins. I wanted to know what was the culprit. This lab revealed I was contaminated and toxic with benzene. I was crushed and very upset. How? why? If you have ever studied benzene it has been known to cause leukemia. It can literally suffocate our blood cell production. You're probably wondering how was I contaminated with benzene? Well, that answer is tricky. I do not know for sure yet, I do remember every evening around 6 PM in Brandon, Florida there would be a black smoke cloud lingering overhead. I heard it was the tire company burning tires after hours when the EPA agency was closed. True or not? Your guess is as good as mine.

One other very important test is D3. It is so essential and it has become more in the highlight due to Covid. It is categorized as a hormone and it regulates over 200 processes in our body. I try to keep my level close to 100 ng/ml in blood serum. It is vital to keep our levels close to 100 ng/ml due to the immune compromise with LGLL.

I was able to quantitatively trace back and gain a better understanding of why, I was the perfect host for LGLL. It took 5 years for me to increase my glutathione level to normal. This is not typical yet, it is for me because I have a gene mutation which causes my body to not absorb glutathione easily. Since then, I have run nutrition labs periodically to maintain strong nutrition levels in my blood and cellular system.

Keep in mind my world was very busy and very stressful during those years, close to my initial diagnoses of LGLL.

3

OUR CHOICES, THEY OFFER

They have a formula. "They" being the University of Virginia, where all the research and data is being collected on LGL. You have your choice of three medications. Are you taking one now? How do you feel?

It is not that easy, and it is not that simple. This leukemia is a rare condition that only 2 percent of the world has been diagnosed with. The official Dr. Thomas Loughran, who has spent his entire career is located at the University of Virginia, and his staff do want to study you. They will fly you to VA and take many tubes of blood, have a consult with you, and fly you back home. They need our data to help them in the study. I think that is a good thing because that is how we progress in science as a whole. This trip will not give you answers, advice on your lifestyle to help you, or give you peace in your heart. Rest assured, it is about getting the data. I was happy to contribute. In June of 2018, while I was in Virginia, I gave him a tip on D3 and the correlating Gene Snp "VDR." I heard later he was advising on a study for D3 and the effects on LGL. *Good! A step in the right direction for others*, I thought. Genes will be discussed in a later chapter. Understanding your genes is valuable, yet keep in mind, "This is not a hereditary condition; it is acquired," as stated by Dr. Thomas Loughran, Jr., University of Virginia.

I have read many of your postings on the Facebook LGL support page, and I am heartbroken because many of you seem lost in a sea of symptoms that just keep getting worse. Sure, you will have a relapse, but it is short-lived, and then your (white blood cell) numbers fluctuate and skyrocket and then your storm is calm again.

I have had to navigate this path myself, I struggled and cried for help, answers, and guidance. That is why I wanted to write this. You do not have to struggle; you just have to rearrange things in your life, make some changes, and do your work.

Every doctor I have spoken to does not want to discuss how it happened. Doctors from Mayo, U of VA, or even my local doctor. If you do not know how it happened then, how are you going to fix or in the medical world go into "remission"?

Think back to a time when you had compounded stress. The perfect storm. The thought that LGL stems from a virus is not too far off, a virus requires a perfect host to attack. This, your genetics, and the perfect storm of stress is the best time for a virus to go into your system and reconfigure the "software of your cells." Ours, it just happens to be in the bone marrow and/or lymphatic where production begins.

Now, if you think about this, it really cannot happen this easily. The body is incredibly sophisticated. It has multiple security levels that this virus has to get through. So here are the perfect conditions. For example, work is stressful; there's a possible death in the family; you live near a power line and a paper mill that excretes toxic fumes; you live near a farm that sprays atrazine on the corn crops, or you recently moved into a new home which off-gases for six to seven years (unless you have super HEPA filtration system, which can reduce it to three to four years). You use commercial deodorant or shampoo hygiene products that have chemicals; you are always rushing from one place to another, whether it be the kids, your elderly parents, etc.; your groceries are more boxed items and not fresh vegetables… Do you get the picture? These are just examples of everyday living.

Your liver becomes congested, chemicals are wreaking havoc, and you are toxic. It is not always a genetic condition or something you can pass on to your children. LGL attacks a perfect host. Think back to where your life was when you think this started. Now, go back at least five to eight years. In your mind, think of where you were and what you were doing. Was your life good, strong, and you were eating healthy and very happy? Or was your life filled with stress, crisis, trauma, and your diet and lifestyle unhealthy?

A perfect host for a virus has high amounts of oxidative stress; emotional, mental, and physical. One or all three are present.

But this is a normal life; it is exactly how everyone around you is living. Eventually, the body starts to have symptoms. By now, you may be thinking about when these symptoms first started, years before you were diagnosed. I hear you; hindsight is 20/20. I feel the same way. If I only knew. Well, you do now, and your children hopefully will hear your story. We can better our future through our children, yet we have to teach them what we are learning.

What Is Your Mind Telling You?

So, here you are going to doctor's visits after doctor's visits, and they take your blood, and it is not getting better—it is getting worse. Your neutrophils are dropping; all you see in the lab report is **LL**. What does this all mean?

Let's take a moment and discuss your labs. Generally, your doctor will run a CBC with a WBC differential, which breaks down the different kinds of white blood cells. This will give him or her an idea of what your immune system is doing or just how vulnerable you are. You must look at your WBC. Is it low or high? The very first sign of an autoimmune is a very low WBC. Yet, chances are, they are high because you have passed the first sign. When you have a chronic autoimmune disorder, which means your body is working in overdrive. It is constantly working, and therefore, you feel fatigued. Knowing your labs can help you but also, hurt you. There were days I felt great when I walked into the doctor's office and after seeing my labs I felt defeated!

There is something psychological about going to your doctor's office. You have an appointment; others know you have an appointment. When you go, the staff has learned who you are and know you, and it becomes almost social! Usually, it is a three- to four-hour ordeal. First, you wait in the lobby, then you are called to give blood, three to four tubes depending on what he or she is checking. For me, we have to keep an eye on my iron/ferritin level. My LGL became an autoimmune hemolysis, which I will explain that later in another chapter. Then you are asked to wait in an exam room. If your office visits are like mine, then you know what I am about to say next...

The doctor enters and tells you your levels are very low. Now, here is the difference. I do not take any of the recommended medication. In all earnest, I did try because I was pressured by family members, but all the meds made me sick, and not feel well, along with the fact that they did not change my lab levels. So, what was the point?

Back in the exam room, the doctor and I discuss alternative therapies. There are none in his wheelhouse, yet, to credit my hematologist, he is trying to think outside the box for me. That is what you need to look for—a doctor who is willing to work for you, network, contact his colleagues, brainstorm, and research.

So, let's go over what the choices of drugs are for LGL. You may be on one of them.

There is a flow sheet from the National Comprehensive Cancer Network. This flow sheet for T-cell Large Granular Lymphocyte Leukemia demonstrates a standard of care for patients following the medical protocol. The initial indication is a unique presentation of lab values from a CBC with a WBC differential. I advise it is vital your labs be evaluated by Dr. Loughran to confirm LGL. The first phase is "wait and see." This condition is about management. If you are symptomatic or there are secondary issues associated with this condition, those are the issues that will be treated. The first line of therapy that they offer is methotrexate, low dose.

The methotrexate drug has been around for over 50 years, the doctors feel confident about prescribing this drug. It does deplete folate and if you have a MTHFR mutation, and folate is not addressed then it can be very harmful short term and long term. Luckily, the doctors at Mayo strongly recommend taking folate 6 hours apart from the med. For me, if I do not have adequate folate because I have a +/- MTHFR Snp, I get a very low mood (depressed). That is why it is critical. Overall, I did not feel well on this med. At first, they prescribed it with a steroid. Again, I felt pressured to take it. The steroid is what the medical profession calls a "miracle drug," I understand. I felt amazing on it. More energy, yet at 3:00 PM every day, I would get this debilitating low-mid back pain. I would have to go lie down and slowly breathe. I could not stand, barely walk, barely breathe—the pain was severe. I explained this to the doctor. I am not sure if they heard me or if they are just numb to our problems. I felt alone. Steroids are not meant to stay on long term, and they will destroy organs in their path. The steroid was short-term, and the methotrexate, I took for 90 days, and I recommend giving it a fair chance. I finished the methotrexate and stopped. Several years later, I tried it again as advised by Mayo, to no avail. It did not change any lab values, except a few of my WBC values went lower. I did not feel good taking the drug. The medication hindered my day-to-day quality of health.

I believe strongly in listening to our bodies. There is an innate intelligence that will give us signs when something needs attention. You just have to tune in and listen.

A second drug is cyclophosphamide +/- corticosteroids. The recommended dose is 50mg daily. I was advised to take this drug. Its biggest job is to destroy T-cells, and they believe it will reset your blood count, yet they do state it causes bladder cancer with long-term use. I discovered that this drug is a derivative of mustard gas in WW1/WW2. It has been known to destroy lymphatic tissue and bone marrow. That just did not seem right for me, or in-alignment of my work to help my body heal.

The third drug is cyclosporine, which is suggested to take your entire lifetime to manage LGL.

It is recommended that a response should be evaluated after four months; the follow-up treatment is to continue on medication or intermittently. According to a study published in bloodjournal.org, 2018, Dr. Loughran stated there is no standard of treatment for LGL patients, although he states the immunosuppressive therapy remains the foundation of treatment, which includes methotrexate (MTX), oral cyclophosamide, and cyclosporine (CyA). This is the core protocol recommended. The great news is, at the University of Virginia, they are conducting many trial studies with peptides. I believe peptides are the next best thing.

4

LGL AND CO-CONDITIONS

So, unless your LGL is causing other conditions, you may not be motivated to work on your health. I encourage you to do so before you develop other conditions. For the rest of us, our motivation is driven by trying to feel better.

The last four years have gone by, and every time I have my labs checked, they are low and indicate how unhealthy I am; it is very discouraging. These low levels can knock one down and make you want to give up and feel hopeless. Choose to live, and choose to live healthily. I ask my patients these questions because the will to live can be very powerful.

I have listened to many of you on the supportive Facebook page for LGL. Many of you talk about other conditions; RA, lupus, skin rashes, migraines, Epstein Barr, Herpes virus… These conditions are in your body for life. A virus in the best situation will go dormant, and this is good because you will be able to live a better life without symptoms. Something like RA can also be symptom-free with the right health protocol. If there are no symptoms, then medication is usually not necessary. As long as you are living a low stress, healthy diet lifestyle.

Keep in mind, the more symptoms you have, the more your body is desperately trying to get your attention. Your body needs nutrition, support, and help. Try not to complicate the LGL with the other conditions. The harder you work on your health, you will minimize the other conditions being expressed. Every day, choose to do something healthy for your body. This will get you one step closer to being healthier in the days ahead. I have found what I do today affects me tomorrow.

5

LGL WITH COVID

We struggle with doing what is right sometimes. Our world does move fast, and there are so many choices.

I was excited because in March of 2021, I was working on 11 weeks since my last blood transfusion going into the twelfth week. My co-condition with LGL is hemolytic anemia. This means my red blood cells are being destroyed too fast, and this causes my hemoglobin to drop down to 5-6. This is very low. For four years, I have been getting blood transfusions every four to five weeks. Dr. Moran said, "If you go seven weeks without needing blood, then you are not dependent." I made up my mind that I was going to go beyond seven weeks. I was tired of getting blood. It takes a whole day of your life, and the iron and ferritin levels increase every time. Along with, Covid being rampant the last place I want to be is in the hospital, the irony of my thoughts. When your iron and ferritin stay high, they will eventually start to damage your organs. Their answer is desferol to chelate the iron. This

Rx is very helpful, yet again, it is a chemical that can cause damage elsewhere in your body. To explain, ferritin is the storage of iron in your body; there is no specific tank or holding place. It is contained in your tissue throughout your body's system.

The desforal chelates the iron—flushes it out—which triggers your body to replenish your iron in the bloodstream from your ferritin. It seems that this is a simple way and effective method. It works for me, for now. This is where you have to weigh out the consequences and make the best choice for yourself. I did notice that my ankles will have edema sometimes after having an IV of desforal. Their remedy is Lasik to stimulate the kidneys to release excess fluid. Taking dandelion herb works just as great, it is a natural diuretic. You can purchase this in a capsule at a health food store or the live greens are sold in the salad department at the grocery store.

About the twelfth week, my clinic/office work was busy. Many folks needed help. New patients requested consults. We had team meetings, and the office kept me with longer hours. Work and life were very busy. I will never forget. The last two patients that week, I decided to be for the first time during COVID a bit relaxed. My consultation was in the office and we sat 6 feet apart. Now, remember I am going on twelve weeks without a blood infusion. Allergy season was in high gear, and I felt a sniffly and slight headache. Allergies, right?

Two days later, I started with a cough, an odd cough. I disregarded it due to allergies season. We were outside, and I did not want to alarm others around me, and I truly wanted to believe I was fine. The symptoms progressed rapidly. I began to double down on my supportive supplements, yet the fever started, and it was unmanageable. The fever reached 105 degrees, and I was delirious. The doctor advised my husband to take me to the hospital immediately. When I was admitted, they ran tests and labs immediately and told me my hemoglobin was a 5.7, and I needed two bags of blood before they could address COVID. I do not remember what happened after that until 10 days later, when they took me off the ventilator. My husband took impeccable notes daily, and he spoke to the nurses twice a day to get updates and advice. Our local primary doctor was prompting him on questions to ask and what the answers mean. My covid story is a book in itself, for now I want to share the wisdom I gained.

My strong advice is always to have another person advocate for you. That person is the second set of ears, or if you are in a crisis, they will be your voice. So have some of those hard discussions with that person about your values and the what if's. They will know how to inform the medical staff, which can truly help you in your care or have you that much closer to being released from the hospital.

For us with LGL, COVID becomes a critical delicate dance. When I was released from the hospital, I needed tons of post-COVID care. It is vital to continue a supportive regimen at least eight weeks to follow up care to avoid relapse.

My colleague came over every other day. She gave me chiropractic care and aromatherapy with key specific essential oils. My body was still in a fight/flight mode. I was told that I was not resting in a coma; I was on a "treadmill," fighting for my life. It took over a week with the help of my colleague for my body to register it was not in danger anymore.

I did not sleep through the night until the tenth day out of the hospital. The fatigue following COVID is ferocious. Much of it has to do with that COVID can recalibrate your heart rate to be in the eighties, nineties, or even 100. My husband took my vitals and checked my O2 levels daily. My heart rate stayed in the nineties for four weeks. Slowly, it has decreased, yet it lingers in the eighties. I have had two blood transfusions since I was discharged. My body is healing, but there were layers of healing that took place.

Post COVID, my life was about pockets of time. My days are scheduled with PT, doctors appointments, desforal drips, and eating. Nutrition along with my supplement protocol is critical to healing. The body needs help, detoxing all the chemicals of IV meds and all the cellular and tissue damage from the virus. Remember, when we are healthy, we are *not* the perfect host for a virus.

I took a month and a half off of work, just to heal and gain my strength back. The time was spent doing just that, and also, reevaluating my work-life balance. There are times in our lives that we do need to regroup, reorganize, and maybe even change our routine.

Here was my post-COVID *protocol supplement support:

Andrographis
Immuneplex
Congaplex
Sesame seed oil
Pneumotrophin PMG
Probiotic
Magnesium
Zinc
D3
Vege nutrition shake daily

Phase 2:
Added methyl folate; glutathione; vitamin E; arginine; multi/mineral; cats claw; burdock, and fish oil.

Stopped the congaplex and the andrographis

*many of these products were from Standard Process

My nutrition was dark leafy greens daily with protein; organic chicken; fish; and grass-fed beef. I used ghee with turmeric daily. This is clarified butter, which is very healing. It is lactose and casein-free. Rebuilding and replenishing were vital to gain my strength and endurance back.

If you are trying hard to prep and cook healthy food, yet find that it is too stressful for you, I recommend Sunbasket and Daily Harvest. These are prepped food companies that use organic ingredients. They are shortcuts without shortcutting your nutrition. Remember, eliminate stress and strive for a work-life balance.

6

ANTI-INFLAMMATORY

There is so much to learn about this virus, yet what is extremely essential is how having LGL and getting COVID can affect you. Having an autoimmune disease makes us more vulnerable. Our immune system is always working and overactive. This alone makes us perfect hosts for this virus. The theory is to calm down the immune system, not to turn it off. The fatigue comes from our bodies working so hard all the time. The labs show just how hard our bodies are working. One of the key components to calming down our immune system is to reduce inflammation. There are two easy, simple items you can add to reduce inflammation; CBD oil and a product from Nutridyn called PRM Resolve.

SPM is pro-resolving modulators that help the body repair when tissue and cells are under attack. The signal molecules are created in your body to end inflammation and repair damage. They are the soldiers that help call in your fighting cells and orchestrate your rehab cells to repair after there have been damaged. These are made by the body, yet when taking ibuprofen or NSAIDS, our body reduces the production of SPMs. Here is the key to SPM's: They are produced in the tissue by immune cells and promote resolution or completion of physical challenges, like stress.

Consider what you eat and how your food can reduce your inflammatory triggers. Here is a list of a few items to consider:

Anti-Inflammatory Foods

An anti-inflammatory diet should include these foods:

Olive oil

Green leafy vegetables, such as spinach, kale, and collards

Nuts, like almonds and walnuts

Fatty fish, like salmon, mackerel, tuna, and sardines

Fruits, such as strawberries, blueberries, cherries, and orange

It's when the body falls into a state of chronic inflammation that big illnesses begin to appear.

Autophagy is very important in reducing inflammation and getting rid of virus cells. This method is achieved through intermittent fasting.

Intermittent fasting is a strong recommendation for LGL. It will reduce other comorbidities, such as diabetes and high cholesterol. Yet for us with LGL, it is another tool for you to stimulate stem cell production and instigate autophagy. Autophagy is the cleansing of destroyed cells that will linger in the body and wreak havoc. Autophagy will help your cells become stronger and healthier, so your body is more resilient to stress. If you have paid close attention, your lab values will fluctuate based upon the level of stress in your lifestyle, which can compromise your immune system. Autophagy will help your body function better. The healthier cells will make you more resilient to stress, inflammation, chronic pain, and disease.

Five Benefits of Autophagy
Gets rid of senescent cells
Improves mitochondrial health
Eliminates viral infected cells**
Reduces cellular apoptosis
Creates stronger and more stress-resilient body and mind

** *Again, another tool for you to dominate your health of having LGL, are intracellular pathogens that impact your cellular system. A supportive immune system place viruses in a dormant state; it will not rid the body of them. Autophagy will remove infected cells and replace them with healthy cells.*

How do you give your body a break? How do you let your body know that it does not have to work so hard?

Well, you can feed your body with highly nutritious food, comfort, low stress, downtime, exercise daily (20 minutes), infrared sauna, slower schedule, ask for help, pray, have others pray, hydrate with clean, filtered water, use all-natural housecleaners, air filter HEPA.

If you have secondary conditions with your LGL, such as RA, keep in mind this is an inflammatory disease. You may have been susceptible genetically to get RA, but it was your lifestyle that dirtied the gene. Clean your gene with every tool you have available: diet; stress-relief techniques; intermittent fasting; infrared sauna; sunlight (D3); proper target nutrients (supplements); and a strong social support system. Keep a watch out for literature coming out on melatonin. It has a bigger value than what we once thought which was just for sleep.

Speaking of genetics, it is very valuable to know and understand who you are genetically. Genes load the gun, but your lifestyle pulls the trigger. For more information on this subject, read *Dirty Genes* by Ben Lynch, ND. There, he will explain more thoroughly how lifestyle "epigenetics" can directly affect your propensity for sickness and disease.

7

RESTORATION FROM THE BOTTOM UP

So many of you have complex other health issues with LGL. If this started as a virus, then what you are experiencing is an autoimmune condition. There are many theories out there about autoimmune. Many indicate it is not curable. I believe you just do the best you can to strengthen your body and not to allow the AI to express itself. AI starts with your gut, from the opening of your mouth to the end of your anus.

Hence, we begin our step-by-step journey.

No Matter What, Heal Your GUT
This takes a lot of mental change because your mind has habits. You have conditioned your mind to live and eat a certain way, whether it came from your upbringing or college years, or just laziness. Your gut lining dictates how you feel. Firstly, to experience happiness and joy, you have to manufacture serotonin, of which 90 percent is made in your gut. If you feel good, you can do anything! True, or true?

The gut becomes damaged over time from birthing forward; vaccines; antibiotics; contaminated food; anesthesia from surgery; stress; overeating; under-eating; etc. The great thing about this is that the gut lining can be fixed. Many nutrients help rebuild the gut lining. For instance, Vitamin A is one nutrient that has powerful cellular replication capabilities.

Gut flora can be properly restored with therapeutic care and probiotics. The products I found to be favorable are from Nutridyn. I used Dynamic GI Restore for two years, five days two scoops, and then I switched to One scoop for two years. This will restore function, give you nutrients, and support digestion overall. I took Spore Probio; 2 capsules with food. It is important to have a very durable probiotic that will sustain heat and stomach acid. I also, take an Immune PRP Pro; 2caps/2x a day, along with my basic nutrition support. Such as, Omega Pure Complete, D3, Vitamin C, Methylfolate, Zinc and Pro-Antho forte. This product is a complete antioxidant.

I believe it is very valuable to test your GI function and so, Genova Labs GI effect comprehensive test is a great stool test for your gut. It is critical to know if you are absorbing your nutritious food, and if not, what is exactly preventing you from absorbing—pathogens, bacteria, fungus, etc. This test will also indicate if you have inflammation, dysbiosis, maldigestion, metabolic imbalance and an infection in your gut. This is probably much more that you have ever thought about your poop. Yet, the more information you have about your own body the better you can take of it.

Keep in mind your body was the perfect host for this condition to go crazy and have a party, so now you approach this as 'enough!' Begin to take back over your home, your body. Think of it this way, it is like coming home after leaving for a weekend and finding wall-to-wall teenagers in your home, drunk, still drinking, or puking everywhere. It will take time to throw them out, clean up, and restore your home to the way you want it. Your body is your home; it is where you live.

How Broken Are You?

If you are like I was, then you are going to need intervention and major nutritional restoration. Firstly, there are many really good nutrition tests that you can help you to know specifically what nutrients and how much you need. Start there. Once you have those results and you have established an Integrative doctor, I suggest you consider IV nutrition, along with a progressive protocol to reduce inflammation, restore cellular nutrition and support your immune system.

Here is what I learned: Your body is a symphony, and so it takes time to absorb and replenish your cells. It will not happen on your watch; the body will delicately and gingerly begin to repair cells, tissue, and organs. Remember this, your body is working machine 24/7. I did not do a detox first. I believe it is vital to get your body stronger first. I was given a two-page protocol of vitamin injections to jumpstart my nutrition. It was daunting, I honestly struggled with my vitamin shots daily—some hurt; some bruised; some I forgot. I was very motivated because I made a choice to myself to get better, but there was something else I was battling. It was several years before I could wrap my brain around what was resisting inside of me. As I said, this is a journey.

EPILOGUE

I have been living with Large Granuloma Leukemia for the last 12 years. Initially, it was easy to just ignore it; I believe they called it "wait and see." I wanted to disregard the diagnosis and live normally. I did struggle with my health. I had huge moments of brain fog, heavy fatigue, and sometimes even exhaustion. It was hard for me to admit I couldn't do a task or a chore. When my health turned for the worse and I needed blood infusions, I was determined to learn everything I could in how to fix this issue. My constant question was, how do I optimize my health? What do I need to do? I have tried many modalities, techniques, supplements, and therapies. Many have really helped, and some helped only a little. This booklet gives you clarity based on my experience of what has helped.

Posturing myself as though I have an autoimmune disease gave me a stronger platform on the decisions I made for my lifestyle. To date, I have almost no symptoms except, every 6 weeks I hear my heart beat in my ear. I know it is time to have my CBC checked. That usually means my hemoglobin is too low. My goal is to reverse the switch. I believe if my body turned the switch on 4 years ago to need blood infusions, why not work really hard to be healthy and maybe just maybe, my body will turn the switch off. I can live with LGLL, I cannot manage the need for blood infusions long term. I am continuously trying to mitigate the damage my body is suffering from the blood infusions. This is my race.

As a thank You for reading my 'How to' Booklet, I am extending to you my resource of target supplements by Nutridyn. Go to www.drsage.nutridyn.com to receive 10% discount. See you on Facebook.